THE PERIOD POSSE
Embracing Change and Empowering Others

Tamara L. Abney

Library of Congress Cataloging – in- Publication Data has been applied for.

Paperback ISBN: 979-8-9885806-9-0
eBook ISBN: 979-8-9885806-8-3

PRINTED IN THE UNITED STATES OF AMERICA.

Cover Image purchased from www.stock.Adobe.com.

Book Publishing Services: Pen Legacy LLC. (www.penlegacy.com)

FIRST EDITION

Dedication

To my dear sons, Aerius and Amari, I hope these pages inspire you to stand as unwavering pillars of support for the women in your lives. Always embrace their dreams, champion their aspirations, and empower them to break free from any barrier society may impose. May you both be the champions of equality and change, building a world where all are respected and heard.

And to you, my beloved husband Aerion, thank you for being the rock upon which our family stands and for supporting me with unwavering dedication from the very beginning of SisterFriend, Inc's journey. Your belief in our cause and tireless encouragement has been instrumental in our success. With you by my side, I have found strength, love, and inspiration to continue this work for the betterment of all.

Table of Content

THE PERIOD POSSE
Embracing Change and Empowering Others

A New Beginning

The shrill sound of the alarm clock pierced through Leigh's dream, yanking her back to reality. Groaning, she slammed her hand on the snooze button before rubbing the sleep from her eyes. Leigh was filled with a sense of hope as she stretched her arms above her head and swung her legs out of bed. It was a brand-new day, and although she couldn't have known it, this day would mark the beginning of an exciting journey.

"Morning, Whiskers," Leigh murmured, stopping to bend over and pet her purring cat before stepping into the tiny kitchen of their cozy apartment in Edmondsville.

This vibrant city was a bustling place filled with diverse communities and endless possibilities, perfect for a passionate and driven thirteen-year-old like Leigh. Her family was tight-knit, always supporting one another's dreams and passions. Andrew, her ten-year-old brother, was no exception.

Tamara L. Abney

With his messy hair sticking up in all directions, Andrew poked his head into the kitchen.

"Hey, Leigh," he yawned. "Are you ready for your track practice?"

"Of course!" she replied, grabbing her sports bag and giving him a quick hug before heading out the door.

* * * * *

The sun beat down on Leigh as she lined up with her teammates at the start of the 400-meter dash. She felt her heart pounding in her chest, adrenaline coursing through her veins as she prepared to take off at the sound of the whistle. With a deep breath, she focused her mind on the race ahead.

Phweeee!

The coach blew the whistle, and Leigh's muscles sprang into action, propelling her forward alongside her teammates. She could feel the wind whipping through her long braids as her legs pumped like well-oiled machines. But then, without warning, she felt a warm sensation between her legs.

"Keep going, Leigh!" shouted her coach from the sidelines. "You're doing great!"

She tried to ignore the sensation, but as she rounded the bend, she looked down and noticed blood on her shorts. Her first period had arrived at the worst possible moment—during the middle of an important track practice.

10

Her pulse quickened even more, and she became lightheaded, feeling faint. Her mind raced with worry. What would her teammates think? Worse yet, what about the boys' team that was watching them run? She didn't want to disappoint anyone, but this wasn't something that could be hidden for long.

"Coach?" Leigh called out hesitantly. "I need to stop."

"Are you okay, Leigh?" her coach asked, concerned by her sudden change of demeanor.

"I'm fine," Leigh replied weakly, trying not to show how embarrassed and vulnerable she felt. "I just need a minute..."

"Where are the bathrooms?" she muttered under her breath, scanning the area with her eyes.

As she looked around for a restroom, Leigh started to feel like maybe it was all too much. Why did this have to happen now? Wasn't being a teenager hard enough already? In that moment, Leigh's confidence faltered, and she wished more than anything that she could just disappear.

Leigh's friend and teammate, Emma, noticed she appeared distracted.

"Leigh, you can tell us if something's wrong," said Emma. "We're here for you."

Leigh looked away, avoiding eye contact as her face burned with embarrassment.

"Thanks, Emma," she whispered. "I just... I think I started my period, and I don't know what to do."

11

Emma's eyes widened with understanding.

"Oh, Leigh," she murmured sympathetically. "Do you have anything with you?"

Leigh shook her head. She felt overwhelmed, not knowing what to expect or how to handle the situation. She was dreading going to Coach Barbara and telling her about her predicament.

Nevertheless, with Emma by her side, Leigh approached Coach Barbara, who had been watching them with concern.

"C-C-Coach," Leigh stammered, "I... I started my period and don't have anything with me."

"Ah, I see," Coach Barbara replied gently. "Well, let's get you taken care of. Girls, can any of you help Leigh out?"

Several teammates nodded and began rummaging through their bags. Leigh couldn't believe her teammates were being so supportive. Despite feeling embarrassed for having to ask them for help, she was thankful they were there for her.

"Go on, take what you need," Coach Barbara said. "We'll wait for you."

Coach Barbara's words filled Leigh with a strange mix of relief and dread. She accepted the supplies, her hands trembling as she carried them to the restroom.

Inside the confines of the stall, Leigh felt completely overwhelmed. How could she not have known this would happen? Why hadn't anyone told her what to expect? She wanted to retreat into herself, but shame kept her rooted in place.

Leigh tried not to look at her teammates as she emerged from the bathroom, but when she met their concerned gazes, something inside her stirred. Was it possible they understood what she was going through? Even if they hadn't experienced it yet, maybe they could still help her make sense of all this.

Leigh took a deep breath and looked up at Coach Barbara, who smiled gently.

"It's a natural part of growing up," her coach said reassuringly.

For a moment, Leigh almost believed it. Then doubt crept in again—doubt about whether she could ever accept this new stage in her life without feeling ashamed.

Despite the discomfort that threatened to overwhelm her, Leigh forced herself to meet Emma's gaze and asked, "What do I need to know?"

As her teammates shared their experiences and advice, Leigh felt torn. On the one hand, she was comforted to know she wasn't alone in this journey, yet she was still embarrassed.

"Leigh!"

The sound of her mother's voice brought her back to the present. She turned to see her mother standing near the track's entrance, looking concerned.

"Mom, I..." Leigh hesitated, unsure how to explain what had happened.

Her heart raced as she wondered if her mother

would be understanding or judgmental.

"Your coach called me," her mother said softly, opening her arms.

Leigh stepped into the embrace. Tears welled in her eyes as she prayed her mother would have all the answers she needed.

"Let's go, sweetie," her mother murmured, guiding her towards the car.

Though Leigh felt relieved at her mother's acceptance, she couldn't help but feel anxious about what would happen next.

As they drove to the store, Leigh listened intently as her mother spoke about menstruation. Despite all the answers her mother provided, Leigh couldn't help but feel scared and overwhelmed by it all.

"Leigh," her mother said, squeezing her hand gently as they walked through the store's aisles. "Remember that you're never alone in this. Your friends, your coach, and I are here for you."

Leigh nodded her understanding but couldn't help but feel a sense of guilt for needing so much support from those around her. No matter how hard she tried to keep up with everything life threw at her as a teenager, sometimes she just didn't have the answers.

As they picked out menstrual pads together, Leigh was filled with gratitude for the love and support of those around her.

* * * * *

A few days later, Leigh and her friend, Ada, were sitting on the grass in the park. The sun was setting, casting a mix of vibrant hues across the sky as well as dark shadows. Leigh had been eager to confide in Ada about her recent experience at track practice and seek her advice.

"Ada, I need to talk to you about something," Leigh began hesitantly, picking at the blades of grass beneath her fingers.

"Of course. What's up?" Ada said, her eyes filled with both confusion and genuine concern at Leigh's sudden look of anxiety.

Leigh took a deep breath before explaining what happened during practice. She described her panic and the help she received from her teammates and coach. Even as she shared this with her friend, Leigh couldn't ignore the embarrassment and fear still lingering inside her.

"Wow, that must've been so scary for you," Ada empathized, placing a comforting hand on Leigh's shoulder. "I remember when I first got my period. It was confusing for me, too, because no one had told me what to expect."

"Really?" Leigh asked, feeling a sense of relief knowing she wasn't alone in the way she felt.

"Absolutely," Ada replied, nodding as she recalled her own experience. "I was at school when it started, and I didn't even realize what was happening until I went to the bathroom. I freaked out and ended up calling my older sister for help."

"Your sister? What did she do?" Leigh questioned, curious about how others had handled the situation when it happened to them.

"She told me to go to the school nurse to get a pad and that she would explain everything to me once I got home."

Ada's expression softened, yet Leigh's reaction made her a little hesitant to delve into more details. Still, she continued.

"My sister told me menstruation is normal and that every girl goes through it. Her explanation helped me feel less alone and scared."

While listening to Ada's story, Leigh felt a strange sense of both understanding and disconnection. Despite feeling slightly embarrassed talking about such a personal matter with her friend, she found comfort in the fact that she wasn't alone, even though her body's changes were initially frightening. At the same time, this newfound knowledge filled her with dread. How could she ever make it through this riddled path of growing up?

"Ada," Leigh said hesitantly, "thank you for sharing. It helps me feel less alone."

"Absolutely," Ada replied warmly. "It's important to support each other, especially when these things can be so confusing. We can learn a lot from one another if we open ourselves up to it."

Leigh nodded, a determined glint in her eyes.

The Power of Friendship

Leigh and her friends decided to meet up by their favorite spot—the ancient oak tree, with its sturdy branches that stretched out like welcoming arms. The girls had spent countless hours sharing secrets and laughter beneath its leafy canopy. Today was no different. However, Leigh had something important to discuss with her friends.

"Hey, guys!" Leigh called out, her voice filled with excitement as she jogged over to the oak tree.

Her long legs easily covered the distance. Having just come from track practice, she wore her usual athletic attire—shorts, a tank top, and sneakers.

"Leigh!" Ada waved, her paint-stained fingers leaving colorful streaks in the air as she beckoned her friend closer.

Ada's artistic spirit showed not only in her clothing choices, which were unique and expressive, but also in her outlook on life. She viewed the world through a creative lens, always seeking beauty in the ordinary.

"Hey, Leigh," Sandi greeted, adjusting her glasses while smiling.

An educated girl with an empathetic heart, Sandi was passionate about creating safe spaces for everyone, regardless of their differences.

"Hi, Leigh," Lena said, her eyes sparkling with curiosity.

Always eager to learn and share knowledge, Lena contributed a wealth of information to every discussion and eagerly embraced opportunities to grow.

"Guys, I want to talk to you about something," Leigh said cautiously, her voice barely above a whisper. "It's kind of personal, but I trust y'all."

Taking a deep breath, Leigh looked each of her friends in the eye before letting the words tumble out.

"I started my period last week," she confessed, her cheeks flushing a delicate shade of pink.

"Wow! That's major," Sandi acknowledged, giving Leigh an empathetic nod. "How do you feel about it?"

"I don't know," Leigh admitted, her eyes filling with tears. "At first, I was scared and confused. My emotions have been all over the place."

"Hey, it's okay," Lena reassured her, placing a comforting hand on Leigh's shoulder. "We're here for you. We'll help you get through this together."

"Thanks, guys," Leigh whispered, wiping away a single tear. "I just...I didn't expect to feel so emotional.

It's like there's this storm inside me that I can't control."

"Leigh, it's completely normal to feel that way," Ada explained gently. "Your body is going through a lot of changes right now, and it's natural for your emotions to be affected, as well."

"Really?" Leigh asked, her voice wavering.

"Definitely," Sandi chimed in. "We'll all experience this...if we haven't already. You're not alone in this."

"I remember learning in health class that we have hormones causing our bodies to adjust to becoming young women, which can cause mood swings," Lena added. "It might take some time, but you'll learn how to manage the changes with your emotions during your period."

"Thank you, guys," Leigh replied sincerely, feeling the weight of her worries beginning to lift. "I don't know what I would do without y'all."

"Besides the emotional changes, what else feels different in your body?" Lena asked, genuinely curious about Leigh's experience.

"Ummm..." Leigh paused, trying to find the words to describe the sensations she had been experiencing. "It's like there's this...heaviness in my lower stomach. Sometimes it feels dull and achy."

"Ah, I've heard about that," Sandi said, nodding. "My mom calls them 'period cramps.' I haven't started mine yet, but my mom says that when I do, I might experience those, too."

"Period cramps can vary from person to person,"

Ada stated. "I remember when I first got mine. The cramps were so bad I could barely walk, but now they're more manageable. You'll find ways to cope, Leigh."

"Okay, that's good to know," Leigh responded, looking at Ada with wide eyes.

It was comforting to Leigh to know there were ways she could feel better.

"Yeah, for sure. Everyone's different, though. My sister barely gets any cramps," Ada continued, offering a reassuring smile.

"Ada's right," Lena agreed. "My older cousin told me some people don't feel any pain during their periods. Lucky them, huh?"

"Have you started yours yet, Lena?" Sandi asked curiously.

"No, not yet. But we learned something in health class. Did you know girls typically start their periods between ages nine and sixteen? So, it could happen to me at any time now," Lena explained, proud of her newfound knowledge.

"Wow! I didn't know that," Sandi admitted, impressed by Lena's information.

"Me neither," Leigh added, grateful for her friend's research. "It makes me feel a little less... weird."

"Hey, you're not weird at all," Sandi reassured her, giving Leigh a playful nudge. "We're all going through this together, remember?"

"Yeah..." Leigh nodded, feeling supported by her

friends. "I guess I just need to get used to the idea that my body is changing, and that's okay."

"Exactly," Ada agreed. "It's important to remember our bodies are amazing. They're capable of so much, and menstruation is part of that."

"Totally," Lena chimed in, her eyes shining with excitement. "It's like we're superheroes or something! We can adapt and grow as our bodies change."

"Superheroes, huh?" Leigh laughed, her spirits lifted by her friend's enthusiasm. "I like the sound of that."

"See? There's no reason to be scared or ashamed," Sandi said, grinning widely. "We've got each other's backs, and we'll face these changes together. Right, girls?"

"Right!" Lena and Ada echoed in unison.

"Thank you, guys," Leigh said, smiling through her lingering uncertainty.

Leigh knew that, with her friends by her side, she would learn to navigate this new stage of her life with grace and confidence. And maybe, just maybe, she could start to see herself as a superhero, too.

Leigh looked around at her friends, each of them with bright smiles on their faces.

"You know what?" she began, tucking a stray hair behind her ear. "Let's make a pact. No matter what happens or how we feel about anything, we'll always be there for each other. We can call ourselves...The Period Posse!"

"Ooh, I like that!" Ada exclaimed, enthusiasm

lighting up her eyes. "The Period Posse. It sounds so powerful!"

"Definitely," Sandi added, nodding her head in agreement. "I mean, there's strength in numbers, right?"

"Right," Leigh affirmed, feeling a rush of excitement course through her veins. "So how do we start learning more about all of this? Any ideas?"

"Books!" Lena suggested instantly, her hand shooting into the air. "We could go to the library and see if they have any books on menstruation. I bet there's tons of information we haven't learned yet."

"Great idea," Ada agreed, pulling a small notebook from her bag. "I'll jot down some key topics we should research. Things like menstrual cycles, hormones, and cramps."

"Let's not forget about pads, tampons, and other menstrual products," Leigh added thoughtfully, her brows furrowing. "There are probably more choices out there than we realize."

"True," Sandi mused, tapping her chin. "I heard some girls use reusable products, like cloth pads or menstrual cups. We should look into those, too."

"Definitely," Ada said, scribbling away in her notebook. "And maybe we can find some videos online that explain things visually. It might be easier to understand some concepts that way."

"Good thinking," Lena praised, her eyes sparkling with curiosity. "This is going to be so much fun!"

The Period Posse

"Alright," Lena announced, clapping her hands together. "Let's get to work, Period Posse!"

"Period Posse!" the others echoed, their voices blending as they stood beneath the oak tree, their newfound sense of purpose shining brightly in their eyes.

As they each went their separate ways, Leigh couldn't help but feel both excitement and worry. There was so much to learn, so many new experiences ahead. But with her friends by her side, she was ready for anything.

"Period Posse," Leigh whispered to herself.

Those words were like a mantra that carried her through the rest of the day. Her thoughts buzzed with ideas, plans, and images of girls just like them—uncertain, scared, and maybe even a little embarrassed. Most importantly, she thought of the strength they would find in coming together.

"Period Posse," she said one last time before drifting off to sleep that night, her dreams filled with the promise of change and sisterhood.

Navigating Challenges

The school hallway buzzed with the chatter of students, their voices echoing off the rows of lockers.

"Alright, Period Posse, let's do this," Leigh said as she glanced at her friends, her voice barely heard above the noise.

The four girls exchanged nods and split up, each on a mission to gather information.

As Leigh strolled through the library, her fingers trailed over the spines of countless books, searching for any resources that could deepen her understanding of menstruation. Eventually, her quest led her to a small section on health. Disappointment washed over her as she examined the lackluster selection. Out of frustration, she plucked an outdated-looking book from the shelf, hoping for a glimmer of enlightenment. However, her hope waned as she flipped through the pages. She didn't find anything helpful. With a sigh, she reluctantly returned the book to its place.

"Hey, Leigh. Any luck?" Lena asked, plopping down next to her with an armful of books.

"Ugh! Not really," Leigh groaned, scrunching up her face. "It's like they want to keep us in the dark about our bodies."

"Tell me about it," Lena chimed in, clearly frustrated. "But guess what I found online on the Cleveland Clinic's website? Did you know menstruation is driven by hormones? And those hormones are chemical messengers in your body. Our pituitary gland, which is found in our brain, and our ovaries, that are part of our reproductive system, make and release certain hormones at certain times during the menstrual cycle."

"Wait, seriously?" Leigh's eyes widened with curiosity. "Spill the tea, Lena! How does the menstrual cycle actually work?"

Lena grinned, ready to enlighten her friend.

"Well, let me break it down for you. According to this article, first we have the menses phase, which is when your uterus lining sheds through your vagina if you're not pregnant. It usually lasts around three to five days, but anywhere from three to seven days is normal. Next is the follicular phase, happening from days six to fourteen. During this time, estrogen levels rise, making your uterus lining grow. Another hormone called FSH also causes follicles in your ovaries to grow. Around days ten to fourteen, one of these follicles releases a mature egg. Then comes ovulation, which usually occurs around day fourteen in a twenty-eight-day cycle. A hormone called LH triggers your ovary to release the egg. Lastly, we have the luteal phase, lasting from about day fifteen to day twenty-eight. The egg travels through your fallopian tubes to your uterus, and progesterone levels rise, preparing your uterus for pregnancy. If the egg isn't fertilized, your hormone levels drop, and your uterus lining sheds during your period. So that's the whole menstrual cycle in a nutshell."

Leigh grinned, absorbing the newfound knowledge.

"I never thought I'd find the menstrual cycle this fascinating. Who knew we had so many hormones?"

Lena shrugged playfully. "Hey, it's all part of being a teenage girl. We're riding these hormonal rollercoasters whether we like it or not!"

Meanwhile, Ada and Sandi approached the school nurse, Ms. Thompson, hoping she could provide some answers. Ms. Thompson welcomed them warmly, her kind eyes reflecting empathy.

"Girls, I wish I could provide more resources for you," she told them. "Unfortunately, the school doesn't prioritize comprehensive menstrual education, and what we do have is minimal."

"Is there anything we can do to change that?" Sandi asked, her voice filled with passion.

"Spread awareness," Ms. Thompson encouraged. "Help your peers understand what's happening to their bodies and that it's normal."

"Thanks, Ms. Thompson," Ada said as they left the nurse's office. "We'll do our best."

Later, the girls reconvened in the cafeteria, sharing what they had learned. Leigh couldn't help but feel disheartened by the lack of resources available. It seemed every new piece of information only led to more confusion.

"Hey, don't worry about it. We'll figure this out together," Sandi reassured her.

As the bell rang, the four friends knew their mission was far from complete, so they all headed back to the library. Since there were few books on the subject, the girls went online.

"Listen to this," Lena called out, her voice cracking with disbelief. "There's something called 'period poverty' that affects people worldwide."

"Period poverty?" Ada echoed, frowning as she leaned closer to Lena's screen. "What does that mean?"

"It means inadequate access to menstrual hygiene products and education," Lena explained while scrolling through an article she found on the website of the nonprofit organization SisterFriend, Inc. "Some people don't have access to sanitary products, washing facilities, or proper waste management."

"Wow," Sandi whispered, her eyes widening. "I never really thought about how lucky we are just to have pads and tampons."

"Exactly," Lena continued, taking charge of the conversation. "We may not have the best resources at school, but at least we have something. There are girls who miss school because they can't afford these products or know how to use them."

Leigh clenched her fists, feeling a surge of anger rise within her. She couldn't understand if this was something so natural—something that happened to every girl—why it was such a struggle for some to have access to menstrual hygiene products. It wasn't fair.

"Okay, this isn't just about our school anymore," Leigh stated firmly. "We need to do something bigger. We need to help those who don't have access to the things we take for granted."

"Do something like what?" Ada asked, her eyes shining with curiosity.

"Maybe we could start a fundraiser or collect donations of sanitary products," Sandi suggested, her tone hopeful.

"Or create educational materials for students in our school and others who might not have the information they need," added Lena.

Leigh nodded, her heart pounding with excitement. They were onto something. With a larger goal in mind, she knew they had the power to make a difference bigger than they had imagined.

Inspiring Advocacy

"Alright, team," Leigh declared as she opened her laptop, "I think we should reach out to SisterFriend, Inc. We need their guidance and support in this fight for menstrual education and advocacy, and they are located in our very own town. I'm drafting the email now."

Leigh's fingers went to work flying across the keyboard.

"Dear SisterFriend, Inc.," she read while typing, "we are a group of thirteen-year-old girls passionate about making a difference in our school, and we would like to learn more about your work in menstrual equity and education..."

"Make sure to mention The Period Posse," Ada reminded her, not looking up from her computer screen.

"Good call, Ada. We want them to know we're serious about this," agreed Sandi thoughtfully.

Lena nodded enthusiastically, her eyes lighting up

at the prospect of learning even more.

"Sent!" Leigh announced triumphantly, pressing the enter key with a flourish.

The four girls exchanged excited glances, their hearts beating with anticipation. They knew they were taking an important step towards making a significant impact in their community.

Within hours, they received a response from SisterFriend, Inc. The girls huddled around Leigh's laptop, reading the message aloud together.

"Hello, Period Posse," Leigh read, her voice brimming with excitement. "Thank you for reaching out to us! At SisterFriend, Inc., we believe in the importance of menstrual equity and providing period products to those in need. Our work involves partnering with schools, shelters, and other organizations to ensure everyone has access to the necessary supplies..."

"Wow, they do so much good," whispered Sandi, her eyes widening with admiration.

"Keep reading, Leigh," urged Lena, her thirst for knowledge not yet quenched. "What else do they do?"

"Additionally, we offer educational workshops and training programs to raise awareness about menstruation and promote a healthy dialogue regarding menstrual health. We would be more than happy to provide guidance and collaborate on your advocacy efforts. In fact, you young ladies should join us at our next workshop..."

"YES!" Ada exclaimed, throwing her arms up in

celebration. "This is exactly what we needed!"

Leigh continued reading the email, picturing the potential impact their partnership could have on their school. She imagined a world where students no longer whispered in shame about periods but openly discussed and supported each other through this natural process.

"Alright, girls," Leigh said, beaming at her friends, "let's get to work. We've got an incredible organization behind us. I'm so glad they agreed to help us. I'm sure we can make a difference with them in our corner."

* * * * *

Leigh's heart raced as she entered the vibrant SisterFriend Educational Workshop. The room hummed with animated conversations, and colorful posters adorned the walls, brimming with valuable information. It was a teenager's dream come true—a treasure trove of knowledge just waiting to be discovered.

"This is going to be so cool," Ada whispered.

Her eyes widened at the array of resources before them as she clutched her sketchbook tight, eager to capture ideas for their own event back at school.

Lena's gaze swept across the room, determination shining in her eyes.

"Let's soak up all the wisdom we can find. We need to bring back ideas to inspire and educate the kids at school. And don't forget; we need to speak with Samantha, the executive director, about partnering on

Tamara L. Abney

an event."

Sandi's grip tightened on her bag, the weight of responsibility settling on her shoulders.

"Absolutely, Lena."

The friends set off, each drawn to different displays and stations like bees buzzing from flower to flower. They immersed themselves in conversations, engaged with passionate activists, and absorbed countless facts and figures. Posters about period poverty, menstrual health, and sustainable hygiene products caught their attention, igniting a fire within their souls.

Leigh furiously jotted down notes, scribbling facts about the global impact of period poverty and the staggering number of individuals affected. She marveled at the innovative solutions showcased, from reusable menstrual cups to community-led initiatives breaking the stigma surrounding menstruation.

Ada's sketchbook became a canvas of inspiration as she captured the powerful stories shared by activists. She depicted colorful illustrations of diverse individuals advocating for menstrual equity, their voices resonating with strength and determination.

Lena delved into conversations with experts, absorbing knowledge about menstrual health education and the importance of breaking down taboos. She scribbled down ideas for engaging workshops and interactive sessions, envisioning a safe space where students could openly discuss menstruation without shame.

34

Sandi gathered brochures and pamphlets, organizing them carefully in her bag, determined to share this wealth of knowledge with their school community. She learned about the different organizations—locally and internationally—working tirelessly to tackle period poverty and their initiatives to provide free menstrual products and promote education.

Leigh couldn't contain her curiosity as she approached a volunteer at one of the tables.

"Hey, do you have any ideas for activities we can organize at our school event?"

The volunteer's face lit up, clearly thrilled to share their knowledge.

"Absolutely! Let me give you a few examples to get your creative juices flowing."

Leigh eagerly accepted the printed list the volunteer produced, scanning it with her eyes.

"Okay, hit me with it!"

The volunteer grinned and started reading off ideas.

"First, you can organize a menstrual health trivia game. Create teams and ask questions about menstrual health, hygiene, and the importance of destigmatizing periods. It's an educational way to test knowledge and debunk myths."

Leigh nodded, picturing her friends eagerly competing while learning at the same time.

"That sounds awesome! I can already imagine how much fun that will be for all."

"Another idea is to host a period product drive," the

volunteer continued. "Encourage students and teachers to donate individually-wrapped period products, like pads and tampons, as well as other essential items like underwear. Then you can distribute them to those in need within your school community."

Leigh's eyes widened, envisioning bins filled to the brim with donations and the joy on the faces of those who would receive the items.

"Yes! We can make a real difference by ensuring everyone has access to the necessary products for FREE."

The volunteer nodded.

"Absolutely," they replied, enthusiasm evident in their voice. "One more idea is to organize a panel discussion on menstrual health. Invite experts, educators, and students to share their experiences, insights, and knowledge about periods. It can be a safe space for open dialogue and provide a platform for breaking taboos."

Leigh's heart fluttered at the thought of the conversations that could unfold.

"That's perfect! We need a space where people feel comfortable discussing menstruation without judgment or embarrassment."

The volunteer smiled, pleased to see Leigh's excitement.

"These are just a few examples, but the possibilities are endless. Get creative, involve your peers, and remember that education and support go hand in hand.

With these activities, you can help create an environment where everyone feels informed and empowered."

"Wow! Thank you so much!" Leigh beamed, thankful for the information and guidance.

She imagined the excitement of her peers as they learned and grew together, breaking down barriers and creating a more inclusive environment.

"Leigh, over here!" Sandi called out, waving her over to where she stood next to Samantha, Executive Director of SisterFriend, Inc.

"Hi, Samantha," Leigh said, extending her hand. "I'm Leigh, and my friends and I are part of a group called The Period Posse. We wanted to talk to you about partnering with us for an event at our school."

"Nice to meet you, Leigh," Samantha responded warmly, shaking her hand. "Sandi has told me about your group's efforts, and I'm impressed by your passion for menstrual education. We'd be honored to work together on an event."

"Really? That's amazing!" Ada exclaimed, joining in on the conversation. "We have so many ideas and can't wait to get started."

"Fantastic! Let's schedule a meeting soon to discuss how we can best support each other," Samantha suggested, exchanging contact information with the girls.

"Thank you, Samantha," Leigh said, grinning from ear to ear. "Together, we'll make a real difference at our school."

As they left the workshop, their minds overflowed with

Tamara L. Abney

new knowledge and inspiration. The Period Posse knew they were one step closer to transforming their school. Pumped and ready to go, they couldn't wait to turn their dreams into reality.

Breaking Barriers, Changing Minds

Inspired by their attendance at the SisterFriend event, they gathered to plan their own Period Party.

Leigh took charge, saying, "Our Period Party is going to be amazing! We need to cover everything about periods—how they work, the products, and the unfairness girls sometimes face."

"Totally!" Sandi exclaimed, remembering her family's past struggle to get period products. "We have to make sure everyone knows that everyone deserves access to period stuff, no matter how much money they have."

Ada flipped through her notes, growing more and more excited.

"Let's make it fun for everyone. And let's not forget about the guys. We want them to have fun and be comfortable, too!"

Lena nodded, glasses sliding down her nose.

Tamara L. Abney

"Teaching guys about periods is important," Ada continued. "We want them to understand what we go through and how they can help us.

"One more thing," Lena said, adding to the conversation as her pen scribbled furiously across the page of her notebook. "Let's not forget that boys can also advocate for menstrual equity. They can join us in raising awareness, challenging stigma, and advocating for better access to period products for all. Boys play an important role in breaking down barriers and creating a more equal society."

Leigh nodded enthusiastically, her long braids swishing behind her.

"Thanks, Lena. Great point. Getting back to event planning. Let's think about how we can collect tampons, pads, menstrual cups—the works. The more options we can provide to our classmates, the better."

Leigh spread out a map of their town on the library floor, a sea of streets and buildings that she hoped would soon be marked with red crosses. Each cross would represent a location where donations for their Period Party could be collected.

Looking up at her friends seated around her in a tight circle, she said, "We need to think hard about where to place our donation boxes. Community centers, local shelters, businesses—let's cover every corner of this town."

"Good idea," Lena chimed in, tapping her pen against her chin as she peered down at the map. "We should also set up an online platform for people who can't make it to these locations. That way, they can directly contribute menstrual products or even monetary donations. I can ask my dad to help with that."

"True," Ada agreed, her fingers running through her long hair as she mulled over Lena's suggestion. "I can ask my brother to create a website and social media page for The Period Posse. We can add the online donation link there and provide updates on our progress.

As her friends brainstormed, Leigh couldn't help but feel a sense of excitement building within her. This was really happening; they were going to make a difference. She glanced down at the map again, her eyes tracing the lines of the streets that connected their town.

"Once we've got our list, we'll reach out to local businesses and organizations," she said determinedly. "We'll ask if they can support our cause by placing donation boxes in their establishments."

"Right," Lena voiced, her gaze focused on the map as she drew red crosses over the potential locations they had identified. "We should also provide them with information about our Period Party and the issue of menstrual equity. That way, they'll understand why this is so important."

"Absolutely," Leigh agreed. "We'll need to create a solid pitch to convince them to support us. But I know we can do it. Together, we're unstoppable."

Tamara L. Abney

"Unstoppable!" Ada echoed, her eyes sparkling.

"Unstoppable!" Sandi and Lena affirmed in unison.

"Alright, then," Leigh said, clapping her hands together to signal the start of their mission. "Let's get to work. But first, let's get the official okay from Principal Stevens."

* * * * *

Leigh's heart thumped in her chest as she stood outside Principal Stevens' office door with The Period Posse gathered around her. She glanced at her friends and took a deep breath before knocking.

"Come in," came the gruff voice from inside.

The door creaked open, revealing Principal Stevens seated behind his desk, hands folded together. His stern gaze bore down on the girls, making Leigh feel like a small, wilting flower under the blazing sun. She swallowed hard, reminding herself they were there for a vital cause.

"Principal Stevens," Leigh began, her voice wavering slightly, "we wanted to discuss our plans for the Period Party with you."

"Ah, yes," he said, his tone dripping with disdain. "I heard about your little project, and frankly, I find it inappropriate for a school event. It's not something we should be promoting."

Leigh felt her cheeks grow hot with anger. She clenched her fists, trying to keep her composure.

"But, sir, it's an important issue that needs to be

addressed–"

"Leigh's right," Sandi interjected, her eyes narrowed. "Did you know girls miss an average of five days of school per year due to a lack of access to menstrual products? It's unfair and affects their education."

"Besides," Lena added, her voice steady, "menstrual products are subject to a luxury tax in many places, labeling them as non-essential items. This perpetuates inequality and makes it harder for those in need to afford them."

"Exactly," Ada chimed in, her hands trembling. "Did you know one out of every four girls has to improvise period protection because they can't afford proper products? It's time to change that."

Principal Stevens leaned back in his chair, his expression unreadable. Leigh could almost hear the gears turning in his head, but it was unclear whether they were working in their favor or against them.

Leigh exchanged glances with the others, and they shared more "did you know" facts about menstrual equity, shedding light on the inequalities and hardships many face.

"Thank you for your time, Principal Stevens," Leigh said. "We hope you can see the importance of our cause and allow us to continue with our plans."

Principal Stevens sighed, tapping his fingers on his desk.

"I must admit, I didn't realize the extent of this issue,"

he admitted grudgingly. "You've indeed presented some compelling evidence."

The Period Posse collectively held their breath, waiting for his final decision.

"Alright," he said at last, "you have my permission to proceed with your Period Party. But..." His gaze sharpened. "...I expect you to keep it tasteful and educational. Nothing inappropriate or disruptive."

"Of course, sir," Leigh assured him, relief washing over her like a tidal wave. "We promise to make it an event that benefits not only our school but also the community."

"Very well." He nodded, dismissing them with a wave of his hand. "Now, get back to class."

As they filed out of Principal Stevens' office, Leigh exchanged excited smiles with her friends, her heart lighter than it had been moments before. They had faced resistance and emerged victoriously. They were one step closer to making their Period Party a reality.

Growth and Milestones

Leigh glanced around the gymnasium, taking in the colorful decorations and the meticulously arranged tables. She could practically feel the excitement and anticipation pulsing through the room. It was just hours until the Period Party would begin, and Leigh felt a surge of pride at how far they had come.

Ada started unrolling a hand-drawn map of the gym with labeled sections for different activities.

"So we've got the educational booths set up along the walls, each covering specific topics about menstruation like myths and facts, hygiene tips, and how different cultures celebrate it," Ada explained.

Lena's eyes lit up with enthusiasm as she chimed in, "We also have the stage area for our health experts, which includes Nurse Thompson and a local gynecologist who has volunteered her time."

"Great! And don't forget the refreshment tables,

which will have snacks and informational pamphlets that attendees can take home with them," Sandi added, beaming.

"Those pamphlets were an excellent idea, Sandi," Leigh praised, grateful for her friend's attention to detail. "What about the menstrual product collection drive? Do we know how it's going?"

Lena checked her phone and smiled. "According to the latest update from the businesses we partnered with, we've collected over five hundred boxes of menstrual products so far! I can't wait to surprise Ms. Thompson with them."

"Wow! That's incredible!" Leigh exclaimed, her heart swelling with pride. "This is all going to make such a difference."

"Definitely," Ada agreed, giving Leigh's shoulder a reassuring squeeze. "But remember, Leigh, this is just the beginning. We're raising awareness and starting conversations. The real change will come when we continue our efforts and make all things menstrual-related a priority in our school."

Leigh nodded, feeling the weight of their mission settle on her shoulders. She knew Ada was right. The Period Party was an essential first step, but there was still much work to be done.

"Okay," Leigh said firmly, addressing her friends with resolve, "let's make today's event one to remember, and let it be just the start."

"Absolutely!" Lena, Sandi, and Ada echoed, their

voices filled with conviction.

After putting the finishing touches on the gym, they were ready to share their knowledge and passion with their peers, and Leigh knew their event would be powerful.

Making a Lasting Impact

The Period Posse flung open the doors.

"Okay, let's welcome our community partners," Leigh said with a determined smile.

"First up, we have the local health clinic," Lena announced as she consulted the list they had created together.

A group of professionals wearing white coats entered the room, carrying pamphlets and informational materials about various health topics for teens.

"Welcome!" Ada exclaimed, helping to direct them where to set up their display. "We have a table right over here for you."

"Thank you so much for inviting us," one of the nurses replied with a warm smile. "It's wonderful to see young people taking charge of their health education."

"Next, we have some representatives from the LGBTQ+ club at school," Sandi said, her eyes lighting up when she spotted their familiar faces. "Hey! We're so happy you could join us."

"Of course!" the club president responded with enthusiasm. "We believe in inclusivity and supporting all students' needs, especially when it comes to something as vital as menstrual health."

As more vendors and student groups arrived, Leigh couldn't help but take a moment to marvel at how far they had come. They were actually doing it—making a difference in their school and community. Her thoughts drifted back to her initial fear about the changes in her body. Now, she was standing at the forefront of a movement at her school that would help countless others just like her.

"Leigh, come check this out!" Ada called, waving her over to the SisterFriend Kits table.

The kits were carefully assembled in brown paper bags, filled with everything someone experiencing a period might need—pads, tampons, and a simple note of encouragement topped off with a sticker with the SisterFriend's logo.

"Wow! These look amazing," she whispered, running her fingers over the neatly packaged kits. "I bet they're going to help a lot of people."

"Definitely," Ada agreed, beaming with satisfaction. "And look, we've got more donations for our menstrual products drive! A group of teachers came together to donate. How cool is that?"

"Really?" Leigh asked, her eyes widening in surprise

as she looked at the growing pile of boxes and packages on the table. "That's incredible! I can't believe how much support we've received."

"Believe it, girl," Sandi replied, her voice full of confidence. "This proves that if you make people aware of the issue, they will understand the need and support. It is really just something most people don't think about."

With all of the vendors and groups set up, Leigh pushed open the double doors of the brightly decorated room, the vibrant colors and empowering images inviting everyone inside. As students and adults alike began streaming in, the lively chatter and laughter filling the space, Leigh felt her heart swell with pride.

"Welcome, everyone!" she called out, her voice ringing clear and strong. "Thank you so much for joining us at our Period Party! We hope today's event will help break the silence and stigma surrounding menstruation and provide valuable resources and information for all."

"Make sure to visit all of our wonderful vendors and student groups," Lena chimed in, gesturing towards the various tables and booths set up around them. "They're here to share their knowledge and expertise with you!"

"Please don't forget to check out our SisterFriend Kits," Ada added, pointing to the display table. "They're free for anyone who needs them."

"Also," Sandi piped up, her eyes twinkling with

enthusiasm, "we're accepting donations of menstrual products for our drive. Every little bit helps!"

As the crowd dispersed, exploring the booths and engaging in conversations about menstrual health, Leigh couldn't help but marvel at how far they had come. Nearby, Principal Stevens observed the bustling room, his previously stern expression softening as he took in the scene before him.

"Leigh," Ada whispered, nudging her gently, "look at this. We did it."

"Yeah," Leigh replied, a smile spreading across her face as she surveyed the room. "We really did."

The Power of Unity

Leigh looked around the room, taking in the diverse crowd. People of all ages, genders, and ethnicities were in attendance, and she couldn't help feeling happy about the turnout. She loved her newfound confidence in helping others understand and embrace the changes happening in their bodies.

As the crowd began to mingle, Leigh spotted Nurse Thompson chatting with a group of students, her warm smile putting everyone at ease. Leigh's parents stood nearby with big smiles on their faces, beaming with pride at their daughter's accomplishments. Seeing these trusted adults supporting their cause only strengthened Leigh's resolve to continue fighting for menstrual equity.

After a few minutes of mingling, Leigh felt a gentle nudge from Lena, signaling that it was time for her to address the attendees. Her heart raced with excitement as she made her way to the podium, feeling the weight of responsibility on her young shoulders.

Tamara L. Abney

"Thank you all for being here today," Leigh began, her voice steady despite her racing pulse. "We stand before you not just as four friends but as advocates for change. Together, we have worked tirelessly to break down barriers, challenge societal norms, and ensure menstrual equity for all."

Leigh paused, allowing her words to sink in. She thought back to her initial fear and confusion when she first experienced her period and how her life had changed since joining The Period Posse.

"Periods are a natural part of life," Leigh continued, "and it's time we stop treating them as something to be ashamed of. Together, we can create an environment where everyone feels supported, understood, and empowered, regardless of their experiences with menstruation."

As she looked out at the crowd, Leigh hoped this event would mark the beginning of a new chapter—one where menstrual equity was no longer a dream but a reality for all.

The applause thundered through the room like a sudden summer storm, and Leigh felt warmth in her chest. She smiled at the encouraging faces before her, their claps filling her heart with happiness.

"Thank you," she said, raising her hands to quiet the crowd. "But it's not just about providing access to menstrual products, although that is crucial." Leigh looked down, remembering her own frantic search for a pad. "It's about fostering education, empathy, and

54

inclusivity. It's about creating a world where no one feels ashamed or limited because of their period."

The audience nodded, their eyes filled with understanding. Leigh saw some people wiping away tears—young and old, male and female—as her words resonated with them. She knew she was making a difference, and it fueled her passion even more.

"Of course, we couldn't have done this without help," Leigh added. "I'd like to take a moment to thank Samantha from SisterFriend for their invaluable mentorship and tireless work in our community."

She gestured towards Samantha, who raised a hand in acknowledgment, receiving a deserved round of applause.

"Your guidance has been instrumental in helping us lead this movement within our school," Leigh told Samantha sincerely, her eyes shining with gratitude.

As Leigh continued to speak, she quickly glanced around the room. The Period Posse had come a long way in a short time, proving that anything is possible when you put your mind, time, and passion into a cause that is personally important to you.

We'll keep fighting until everyone has the support and resources they need, she promised herself silently, her resolve unwavering.

Throughout her speech, Leigh could feel the energy in the room growing, as if each person present was absorbing her message and ready to carry it out into the world.

Together, we can break down barriers and change lives, she thought, her eyes meeting those of the others on stage with her.

As Leigh stepped away from the podium, she felt a surge of pride and accomplishment as she rejoined her fellow Period Posse members on stage. Sandi, Lena, and Ada beamed at her, their eyes shining with admiration for their determined and passionate leader.

"Great job, Leigh," Ada whispered, giving her a quick hug. "That was amazing."

"Thanks," Leigh replied, her hand trembling with excitement. "I couldn't have done it without all of you."

"Leigh! Sandi! Lena! Ada!" shouted a familiar voice from the crowd.

It was Nurse Thompson, her arms outstretched in a gesture of congratulations. The girls gathered around her eagerly, basking in the warmth of her praise.

"You young ladies are doing incredible work. It's an honor to see you grow and make such a significant impact in such a short timeframe. Keep it up!"

"Thank you so much, Nurse Thompson," Leigh responded, touched by her words. "We appreciate your support more than you know."

"Alright, everyone, let's capture this moment!" called the school photographer, motioning for them to pose together.

The girls huddled close, smiling brightly as the camera flashed.

"Say 'menstrual equity'!" Lena quipped, eliciting

laughter from the group.

"Menstrual equity!" they echoed in unison, their voices strong and confident.

As the attendees continued mingling, several approached The Period Posse. The girls took the opportunity to ask each attendee to sign petitions to get free menstrual products in the school's restroom. One woman, a mother with a teenage daughter, looked particularly moved as she spoke with Leigh.

"Your speech was so inspiring," she told Leigh earnestly. "I've signed the petition, and I promise to talk to my daughter about everything you discussed today. It's time we break the stigma surrounding menstruation."

"Thank you," Leigh replied, her heart swelling with gratitude. *This is what it's all about,* she thought. *Changing minds and making a difference.*

"Excuse me, ladies," said a reporter from the local news station, microphone in hand. "May I ask you a few questions about your initiative?"

"Of course!" Sandi replied enthusiastically, stepping forward to answer on behalf of the group.

As Sandi spoke confidently to the reporter, she couldn't help but feel a sense of awe at their accomplishment. It had taken time, effort, and some convincing, but they were finally seeing the fruits of their labor.

The buzz of the event continued, with people animatedly discussing their experiences and supporting The Period Posse's cause. Leigh was in the midst of a conversation when Principal Stevens approached her with his phone in his hand. She glanced at the screen, seeing an unknown number on it.

"Excuse me," she said to the group, stepping aside to take the call. "Hello?"

"Hi, is this Leigh?" a friendly voice asked on the other end of the line.

"Yes, speaking," she replied, trying to place the unfamiliar voice.

"Leigh, my name is Assemblywoman Rodriguez. I'm calling to congratulate you and your friends on the incredible work you're doing with The Period Posse. Principal Stevens has told me about your event centered around menstrual equity, and I wanted to personally commend you for your passion and dedication."

Leigh's eyes widened with surprise, her heart racing with excitement. A government official had taken notice of their efforts. This was a significant step forward!

"Th-thank you, Assemblywoman Rodriguez!" she stammered, her mind racing. *This could be huge,* she thought as her heart pounded in her chest.

"I'd like to extend an invitation to meet with me next week at my office. I believe there's potential for important legislation to support your cause," Assemblywoman Rodriguez continued, her tone encouraging.

"Wow! Yes, absolutely. We would be honored to meet with you," Leigh replied, her voice shaking with emotion.

This was beyond anything they had ever dreamed of—a chance to make a real, lasting difference.

"Excellent. My assistant will send you an email with all the details. Once again, congratulations on your success. I look forward to our meeting."

"Thank you, Assemblywoman Rodriguez. We're truly grateful for this opportunity," Leigh said, her voice firm with resolution.

As she hung up the phone, she felt even more proud of the work they had done so far.

"Hey!" she called out to her friends, waving them over. "You won't believe this! We just got a call from Assemblywoman Rodriguez. She wants to meet with us to discuss potential legislation supporting menstrual equity!"

Excited, Ada's eyes lit up with excitement, while Lena's jaw dropped in shock. Sandi couldn't help but let out a squeal of joy as they exchanged high-fives, their spirits soaring.

"Can you believe it?" Leigh whispered to herself, still processing the enormity of the situation. *This is our chance to make real change on a larger scale,* she realized, feeling both humbled and empowered by the opportunity before them.

As they celebrated, Leigh couldn't help but think about the countless individuals who would benefit from a world more understanding and supportive of menstrual health.

Beyond the Period Posse

The day after their successful event, they were still buzzing with energy. Leigh, Sandi, Lena, and Ada couldn't help but smile as they recounted the highlights of the event while sprawled across Leigh's bedroom floor.

"Can you believe how many people showed up?" Sandi enthused, her eyes twinkling. "And all the donations we collected!"

Leigh nodded, feeling a swell of pride. "I know, right? I can't wait to see what else we can accomplish."

"Speaking of which," Lena chimed in, pushing her glasses up her nose and flipping open her notebook. "We've got that trip to The Capitol next week. Are we ready for it?"

Ada grinned. "Definitely. Our presentation is strong, and our message is clear. We just need to make sure we stay focused and don't let nerves get the best of us."

"Absolutely," Leigh agreed, her heart pounding at the thought of standing before lawmakers and sharing their advocacy idea. "But first, let's take a moment to celebrate our success."

They clinked their soda cans together, savoring the sweet taste of victory.

* * * * *

A week later, Principal Stevens and the girls found themselves navigating the bustling halls of the Capitol Building, clutching their carefully prepared presentation materials. Their hearts raced as they approached each legislator's office, determined to make their voices heard.

"Remember," Leigh whispered to her friends, her palms sweaty, "we're doing this for everyone who has been held back by their period. We can do this."

"Right," Lena affirmed, adjusting her grip on her stack of research papers. "Let's go change some minds."

As the doors opened and closed behind them, the girls delivered their passionate speeches, the fire in their eyes impossible to ignore. They spoke about the need for menstrual equity and how it affected their peers, their words echoing through the hallowed halls.

"Thank you for your time," Sandi said as they exited the final office. Her voice was steady, but her hands trembled from her nervousness.

"Whew," Ada sighed, tucking a loose strand of hair

behind her ear. "That was intense, but I think we really got through to some of them."

"Definitely," Lena concurred, flipping through her notes. "We've made some strong connections today. Our journey is far from over, but we've taken a huge step forward."

"Agreed," Leigh added, feeling a renewed sense of purpose surging through her veins. "This is just the beginning for The Period Posse. We're not going to stop until everyone has access to the resources they need."

The sun dipped low in the sky, casting a warm shadow on the steps of the Capitol Building where Leigh, Sandi, Lena, and Ada sat, their legs dangling over the edge. They watched as people hurried by, oblivious to the four advocates who had just made their voices heard.

"Can you believe we did it?" Leigh asked, her voice tinged with amazement. She ran her fingers through her hair, which was still slightly damp from the effort of their presentations.

Sandi grinned, her green eyes sparkling. "I knew we could. We're The Period Posse, after all."

Turning back to her friends, Leigh said, "We're not just advocates. We're leaders, bound together by this mission and our friendship. We've come so far already, and I know we'll go even further."

"Absolutely," Sandi agreed. "And we won't stop until menstrual equity is a reality.

"Right," Lena added. "We'll keep working until every school, every community has the resources and support they need."

"Alright," Leigh said, "let's get back to work."

* * * * *

Two weeks later, Leigh's heart raced as she addressed an auditorium filled with students, the microphone in her hand slightly shaking.

"Thank you all for coming today," she said, her voice steady despite her nerves. "We're here to talk about something that affects every girl in this room— periods. Periods are a natural part of life," Leigh explained, remembering her own fears and hesitations when she first started her period. "Our goal is to ensure everyone has access to the information and supplies they need to manage their periods confidently."

As the girls took turns sharing their experiences and stories, the faces in the crowd grew more engaged. They could see the spark of understanding ignite within the minds of their peers, fueling their passion to make a change.

"Starting today, we're partnering with other schools to create clubs like The Period Posse," Lena announced, "Together, we can break down barriers and improve the lives of countless young people."

"Of course," Ada chimed in, "our journey won't be easy. We'll face obstacles and setbacks along the way. But we're committed to this cause and won't give up until students have access to the menstrual products and educational resources they need."

Leigh nodded, her thoughts echoing Ada's sentiment.

As they wrapped up the meeting and began answering questions from the audience, Leigh felt a renewed sense of purpose.

They had made an impact, but there was still so much work to be done. Leigh felt more determined than ever to continue their advocacy efforts, host more informational meetings, and partner with other schools to start similar clubs.

As Leigh looked into the eyes of her friends, she saw their shared commitment reflecting back at her. They were united, bound by the unbreakable ties forged through their advocacy journey.

Leigh took a deep breath, her voice steady and filled with determination as she spoke her final words: "We may be young, but we're capable of creating real change. Let's keep raising our voices, breaking the silence, and fighting for a world where menstruation is no longer a barrier but a badge of strength. Together, we can make menstrual equity a reality."

The crowd erupted into applause, and Leigh felt a surge of pride and hope fill her heart. This was just the beginning of their journey, and she knew that as long as The Period Posse stood united, their impact would continue to grow. They were warriors of change, fighting for a future where no girl would be held back by her period.

With that thought, Leigh stepped off the stage, ready to conquer the challenges that lay ahead, together with her sisters in arms.

About the Author

Tamara Abney is a passionate advocate for menstrual equity and the Founder and Executive Director of SisterFriend, Inc., a Pittsburgh, Pennsylvania-based non-profit organization. Through SisterFriend, Inc's tireless efforts, countless individuals have been provided with essential menstrual products and access to accurate information, breaking down barriers and empowering communities.

With her debut book, "The Period Posse: Embracing Change and Empowering Others," Tamara brings her expertise and dedication to empowering young girls and adolescents, parents and caregivers, educators, and school administrators to advocate for menstrual equity in their schools and communities.

Tamara's writing is inspired by her belief in the power of young voices to break stigmas, embrace knowledge, and drive positive change. Through "The Period Posse: Embracing Change and Empowering Others," she weaves a heartwarming tale of friendship, growth, and resilience, empowering readers to embrace their bodies and menstrual journey with confidence.

As a sought-after speaker and thought leader, Tamara is frequently invited to share her expertise and insights at conferences, seminars, and educational institutions. Her thought-provoking discussions inspire audiences to challenge the status quo, break down taboos, and work towards a more equitable and inclusive society.

Tamara resides with her husband, Aerion, and their two sons, Aerius and Amari. She balances her devoted wife and mother roles with her passion for professional development, health advocacy, and community service.

Connect with Tamara and join the movement for menstrual equity by visiting SisterFriend, Inc's website at www.sisterfriend.org and following them on social media @sisterfriendorg or at her personal website www.tamaraabney.com. Also, follow her on social media @tamaraabney.

Embrace the power of knowledge, and together, let's break barriers, challenge norms, and empower the next generation for a brighter and more equitable future.

www.ingramcontent.com/pod-product-compliance
Lightning Source LLC
Chambersburg PA
CBHW060257030426
42335CB00014B/1745